Accept and Celebrate

Embracing Your True Sexuality

Jason Betz

Table of Contents

INTRODUCTION

The book 'Accept and Celebrate: Embracing Your True Sexuality' is an exploration of understanding, accepting, and celebrating women's as well as men's sexuality. A groundbreaking book that challenges the traditional norms of sexuality and encourages readers to embrace their true selves.

This book will provide readers with insight into their unique pleasure pathways and an understanding of their sexual desires. It equally provides a comprehensive guide to understanding and accepting one's sexuality, regardless of gender or sexual orientation through scientific research.

It will also provide readers with practical advice on how to create a safe and supportive environment to explore their sexuality. The book will cover topics such as understanding hormones and pleasure pathways, body image and self-esteem, the influence of culture, communication, and exploring sexuality without shame. It will also guide how to cultivate a positive sexual self-image and how to celebrate one's true sexuality.

'Accept and Celebrate' empowers readers to explore their sexuality and live a fulfilling life free of shame and judgment. This book is a must-read for anyone looking to break free from societal constraints and embrace their authentic self.

CHAPTER ONE

Introduction to Women's Sexuality

Women's sexuality is an often overlooked and misunderstood subject. Even though women's sexuality has become more accepted in recent years, there are still a lot of misconceptions about what it means to be a sexually liberated woman. Women's sexuality is not just about having sex but also about exploring, accepting, and celebrating one's own body and desires.

It is important to remember that women's sexuality is complex and individual. Every woman is different and there is no one-size-fits-all approach to exploring and accepting one's sexuality. That is why it is important to create a safe and supportive environment to explore, accept and celebrate one's sexuality.

It is also important to remember that the sexuality of women should not be judged or shamed. Everybody have the right to explore their sexuality without fear of judgment and should be empowered to do so.

Women's sexuality should be celebrated and embraced, allowing women to explore and accept their desires without shame.

Women's sexuality is a complex and multifaceted topic that has been studied and explored for centuries. It encompasses a wide range of factors, including physical, emotional, psychological, and cultural influences. Understanding and embracing women's sexuality is crucial for promoting sexual health, gender equality, and overall well-being.

From reproductive health to sexual desire, pleasure, and satisfaction, women's sexuality is a vital aspect of their lives. However, societal norms, cultural taboos, and misinformation often lead to shame, guilt, and confusion around women's sexuality. As such, it is essential to create a safe and inclusive space to discuss and explore women's sexuality, free from judgment and stigma.

With the right knowledge, support, and resources, women can reclaim their sexual agency, explore their desires, and experience a fulfilling and satisfying sex life.

In recent years, there has been a growing awareness of the importance of women's sexuality and the need to prioritize it in healthcare, education, and public discourse.

Women's sexuality is not just about reproduction but involves emotional connections, self-expression, and personal growth. It is a vital aspect of their overall health and well-being, and it is essential to recognize and address the unique challenges and experiences that women face in this area.

Empowering women to understand and embrace their sexuality can lead to increased confidence, self-awareness, and better relationships. It can also promote gender equality by breaking down societal barriers and challenging harmful stereotypes.

Women's sexuality is a dynamic and complex phenomenon that deserves to be celebrated, respected, and explored. By promoting a culture of openness, acceptance, and inclusivity, we can create a world where women's sexuality is valued and celebrated.

CHAPTER TWO

Understanding Hormones and the Unique Pleasure Pathways for Women

Women have unique pleasure pathways due to their hormones, and understanding them can be the key to unlocking amazing sexual experiences and satisfaction. The hormone estrogen is responsible for a range of pleasurable sensations in women, ranging from lubrication of the vagina to deep arousal. Estrogen plays a role in the neurotransmitter and nerve pathways in the brain, and it plays a role in vaginal sensitivity. Testosterone is directly linked to sexual arousal, and it is responsible for muscle and bone strength, energy, and libido.

Oxytocin, often referred to as the "love hormone", is important for intimate relationships and sexual pleasure. Produced in the hypothalamus, this hormone helps build trust and attachment, and it can help women reach orgasm. Finally, dopamine is responsible for arousal, pleasure, motivation, and reward. It is released when women experience pleasure, and it has been found to increase the intensity of orgasms in women.

Understanding hormones and the unique pleasure pathways for women is key to experiencing sexual satisfaction, as hormones can play a big role in a woman's arousal and pleasure. By understanding how hormones influence the body, women can take steps to ensure their sexual experiences are as pleasurable as possible.

The clitoris is an important part of sexual pleasure for women, and it contains more than 8,000 nerve endings. It is located at the top of the vulva and is often referred to as the "pleasure center." When aroused, the clitoris becomes engorged with blood, making it more sensitive to stimulation.

The G-spot is located on the front wall of the vagina, and it can be a powerful source of pleasure for women. When stimulated, the G-spot can lead to intense orgasms and even female ejaculation. Experimenting with different kinds of stimulation, such as direct pressure, can help women discover what gives them the most pleasure.

The anal sphincter is also a source of pleasure for many women, although it can be difficult to access. Toys and lubricants can help make the experience more comfortable and enjoyable.

The breasts are often overlooked as a source of pleasure. Stimulating the breasts can lead to increased arousal and pleasure for many women.

Hormone replacement therapy can be used to treat sexual dysfunction in women caused by hormonal imbalances, and exploring different forms of stimulation, such as clitoral and G-spot stimulation, can lead to more intense orgasms.

It is also important to note that sexual pleasure and desire can vary widely among women and that there is no one-size-fits-all approach to sexual pleasure. Encouraging open communication with sexual partners, exploring different forms of sexual expression, and prioritizing self-care and sexual health can all contribute to a fulfilling and satisfying sex life for women.

It is essential to understand that sexual pleasure and desire can be impacted by various factors, including stress, medication, and medical conditions. Chronic illnesses such as diabetes and cardiovascular disease can affect sexual function, while medications such as antidepressants and antihistamines can cause sexual dysfunction. Additionally, psychological factors such as anxiety and depression can affect sexual desire and function. It is crucial to address these underlying issues to promote sexual health and well-being.

Education and awareness about women's sexuality and pleasure are also critical in promoting gender equality and reducing stigma and shame around sexual expression. Unfortunately, women's sexuality has been stigmatized and suppressed in many cultures, leading to a lack of knowledge and understanding about sexual health and pleasure. It is crucial to promote education and awareness about women's sexual health in schools, universities, and healthcare settings to empower women to take control of their sexual health and well-being.

In conclusion, understanding hormones and the unique pleasure pathways for women is crucial in promoting sexual health and well-being. Women's sexuality is a complex and dynamic phenomenon that deserves to be celebrated and respected. By promoting education, awareness, and open communication about women's sexual health and pleasure, we can create a world where women are valued and celebrated, leading to more fulfilling and satisfying sex lives for women.

CHAPTER THREE

Body Image and Self-Esteem

Body image and self-esteem are closely interconnected, as how we perceive our physical appearance can significantly affect our self-worth and confidence. Body image refers to how we see ourselves physically, including our size, shape, and appearance. On the other hand, self-esteem refers to our self-respect and self-confidence.

Negative body image is a prevalent issue, particularly among women, and can lead to low self-esteem and a range of mental health issues such as depression and anxiety. The media often promotes an unrealistic and unattainable standard of beauty that can create feelings of inadequacy and self-doubt in those who do not fit into these narrow beauty ideals.

It is crucial to promote a positive body image and self-esteem, as it can have a significant impact on our mental and emotional well-being.

Here are some strategies that can help improve body image and self-esteem:

- **Take care of yourself**: Engage in activities that encourage self-care, such as exercise, healthy diet and enough sleep. Taking care of your physical health can help you feel better about your body and improve your overall well-being.

- **Surround yourself with a positive energy**: Surround yourself with people who build you up and support you. Avoid toxic relationships and environments that promote negative self-talk and criticism.

- **Challenge negative thoughts**: When you have negative thoughts about your body, challenge them by focusing on positive attributes and accomplishments. Practice gratitude and self-compassion to help shift your focus away from negative self-talk.

- **Embrace diversity**: Celebrate diversity in all its forms, including differences in body size, shape, and appearance. Recognize that beauty comes in all shapes and sizes and that there is no one "perfect" body type.

- **Seek professional help**: If negative body image and low self-esteem are affecting your daily life and mental health, seek professional help from a therapist or counselor. They can provide support and guidance in developing healthy habits and improving self-esteem.

In addition to the strategies mentioned above, it is essential to recognize that body image and self-esteem are not solely based on physical appearance. Our relationships, accomplishments, and experiences also play a significant role in our overall sense of self-worth and confidence.

Therefore, it is crucial to focus on developing a positive and healthy relationship with oneself. This means treating yourself with kindness and respect, setting realistic goals and expectations, and recognizing your strengths and weaknesses.

Another important factor in improving body image and self-esteem is avoiding comparing oneself to others. Comparing oneself to others can lead to feelings of inadequacy and self-doubt, as everyone's journey is unique. Instead, focus on your progress and accomplishments and recognize that there is no one "right" way to look or be.

Overall, improving body image and self-esteem requires patience, self-compassion, and a willingness to challenge negative thoughts and behaviors. By adopting a positive and healthy mindset and focusing on self-love and acceptance, we can improve our mental and emotional well-being and live a more fulfilling and confident life.

In conclusion, promoting a positive body image and self-esteem is crucial for our mental and emotional well-being. By practicing self-care, focusing on positivity, challenging negative thoughts, embracing diversity, and seeking professional help, we can improve our body image and self-esteem, leading to a more fulfilling and confident life.

CHAPTER FOUR

Cultural Influences and Communication

Culture plays an essential role in communication, as it shapes how individuals perceive and interpret messages. Communication is not solely about the transmission of information, but also about the creation of meaning and understanding between individuals.

Cultural influences affect communication in various ways, including language, nonverbal communication, and social norms. Language is one of the most significant cultural influences on communication, as it shapes how individuals express themselves and interpret messages. For example, some cultures place a strong emphasis on indirect communication, while others prioritize direct communication.

Nonverbal communication, such as body language and facial expressions, also varies across cultures. For example, in some cultures, avoiding eye contact is a sign of respect, while in others; it is seen as a sign of dishonesty.

Culture also affects communication in terms of power dynamics. For example, in some cultures, there is a strong emphasis on hierarchy and respect for authority figures, while in others; there is more emphasis on equality and collaboration. These power dynamics can affect how individuals communicate with one another and can lead to misunderstandings and conflicts.

Social norms, such as values, beliefs, and customs, also affect communication. For example, in some cultures, interrupting someone during a conversation is considered rude, while in others, it is seen as a sign of active listening.

Moreover, cultural influences also shape how individuals express emotions and handle conflict. In some cultures, expressing emotions openly is encouraged, while in others, it is seen as a sign of weakness. Similarly, in some cultures, conflict is seen as a natural part of communication and is addressed directly, while in others, conflict is avoided at all costs.

To communicate effectively across cultures, it is crucial to understand cultural influences and differences in communication and adapt one's communication style accordingly to avoid misunderstandings and misinterpretations.

Here are some strategies that can help improve communication across cultures:

- Be open-minded:

Be open to learning about different cultures and their communication styles. Avoid making assumptions or judgments based on one's cultural background.

- Listen actively:

Listen carefully to the other person and try to understand their perspective. Ask questions and clarify any misunderstandings to ensure that you are on the same page.

- Be respectful:

Show respect for the other person's cultural background and communication style. Avoid imposing your cultural norms or expectations on them.

- Adapt to the situation:

Adapt your communication style to fit the situation and the cultural context. For example, if you are communicating with someone from a culture that values indirect communication, you may need to be more attentive to nonverbal cues.

- Seek feedback:

Seek feedback from the other person to ensure that you are communicating effectively. Ask them if they understand your message and if there is anything, you can do to improve communication.

Other additional strategies that can help are

- Avoid stereotypes:

Avoid making assumptions about individuals based on their cultural background. Instead, focus on getting to know them as individuals and understanding their unique communication styles.

- Be patient:

Communication across cultures can take more time and effort than communication within one's own culture. Be patient and allow for extra time for clarification and understanding.

- Use simple language:

When communicating with individuals whose first language is not the same as yours, use simple language and avoid idioms or slang.

- Be aware of nonverbal cues:

Pay attention to nonverbal cues such as facial expressions and body language, as these can vary across cultures and can affect how messages are interpreted.

- Seek out cultural training:

Consider taking a cultural training course or working with a cultural mentor to improve your cross-cultural communication skills.

In conclusion, cultural influences play a significant role in communication, and it is essential to understand and respect them to communicate effectively across cultures. By adopting an open-minded, respectful, and adaptable approach, individuals can improve their communication skills and build stronger relationships with people from different cultural backgrounds.

CHAPTER FIVE

Exploring Your Sexuality without Shame or Fear

Sexuality is a complex and multifaceted aspect of our lives and exploring it can be a challenging and sometimes daunting experience. However, it is essential to understand that there is no shame or fear in exploring your sexuality, as it is a natural and normal part of being human.

To begin exploring your sexuality, it is crucial to start by understanding your desires and interests. Take the time to reflect on what turns you on, what arouses you, and what you find pleasurable. This self-exploration can take many forms, from experimenting with different fantasies, exploring your body through masturbation, or trying out new sexual experiences with a partner.

It is also important to recognize that sexuality is a personal and individual experience, and there is no right or wrong way to explore it. What may work for one person may not be the same for another, and that is perfectly okay. The key is to be open-minded, curious, and respectful of your boundaries and those of others.

Another critical aspect of exploring your sexuality is communicating with your partner(s) openly and honestly. Whether you are in a committed relationship or engaging in casual encounters, it is essential to discuss your desires, boundaries, and expectations. This communication can ensure that everyone involved feels comfortable and respected and can lead to a more satisfying sexual experience for all parties.

It is important to seek out resources and support if needed. This can include talking to a therapist, joining a support group, or seeking out educational materials on sexuality. Remember, exploring your sexuality should be a positive and empowering experience, and there is no shame in seeking out help or guidance along the way.

When it comes to exploring your sexuality, it is important to keep in mind that everyone's journey is different, and there is no "right" or "wrong" way to approach it. Some people may choose to explore their sexuality through pornography, while others may prefer to read books or attend workshops. Some may be interested in exploring their sexuality with multiple partners or engaging in kink while others may prefer methods that are more traditional.

Whatever your approach, it is important to prioritize consent and safety. This means being clear and open about your boundaries, using protection during sex, and respecting your partner's boundaries as well. It is also crucial to educate yourself about sexually transmitted infections and other risks associated with sexual activity and to take steps to protect yourself and your partners.

While exploring your sexuality can be a liberating and fulfilling experience, it is also important to remember that it is not a requirement. Some people may choose to abstain from sex altogether, or may not feel comfortable exploring their sexuality for personal or cultural reasons. Whatever your choice, it is important to respect your boundaries and make decisions that feel right for you.

In conclusion, exploring your sexuality is a natural and normal part of being human, and there is no shame or fear in doing so. By taking the time to understand your desires, communicating openly with your partner(s), and seeking out resources and support when needed, you can embark on a fulfilling and enjoyable journey of sexual exploration.

CHAPTER SIX

Creating a Safe and Comfortable Sexual Environment

Creating a safe and comfortable sexual environment is essential for enjoyable and fulfilling sexual experiences.

Here are some points for creating such conditions:

Communication

The most important thing to keep in mind when it comes to creating a safe and comfortable sexual environment is communication. You should be clear and open with your partner about your boundaries, desires, and expectations. Make sure you both have a mutual understanding of what you are comfortable with and what you are not.
Prioritize communication above all else, it is the cornerstone of any successful relationship!

Consent

Consent is the paramount part of any sexual relationship. You and your partner must be on the same page when it comes to giving and receiving consent, so make sure that you are both enthusiastic about what is happening before proceeding with anything else. Consent should be ongoing throughout a sexual experience, not just at the beginning or end of the act. In addition, it should always be freely given--if someone is not comfortable with something that is happening during sex, they have every right to say no!

Privacy

The first step to creating a safe and comfortable sexual environment is to make sure you have a private space where you can engage in sexual activity without interruption or fear of being seen or heard. This may sound obvious, but it is important enough that we are going to say it again; Prioritize privacy!

If there are people around your house who might be able to see into your bedroom window at night, if there is a chance they will hear what is going on inside your room by pressing their ears against the wall (or even just knocking on the door), then this is not an ideal location for sex.

The same goes for other potential interruptions like pets--you do not want them jumping up onto the bed at an awkward moment or barking incessantly outside the door while you are trying to get down with someone else.

Protection

You should have access to condoms, dental dams, and other protection methods. If you are not sure what these are or how to use them, ask your healthcare provider or visit a local sexual health clinic for more information.

Use protection consistently and correctly to prevent sexually transmitted infections (STIs) and unwanted pregnancy. Prioritize protection over pleasure; it is better for both of you if you do not have an STI or get pregnant!

Comfort

Before you even get to the fun part, you should make sure that both of you are comfortable with the setting. The lighting and temperature should be just right, and there should not be any distractions--no kids running around or pets barking in the background. If these things are not taken care of beforehand, they could easily ruin an otherwise great sexual experience by distracting one or both partners from focusing on each other's needs.

Prioritize comfort above all else when planning out your sexual encounters; this means making sure that everything from clothing choices to position preferences are agreed upon ahead of time so no one feels pressured into doing something he or she doesn't want to do just because it seems like "the thing" at that moment in time (or worse yet: because someone else thinks he or she should).

Trust

Make sure you and your partner trust each other and feel safe expressing your desires and boundaries.

Prioritize trust. Trust is the foundation of any healthy sexual relationship, so make it a priority to build up this quality in yourself and others before getting started with sex play.

Respect
Respect is one of the most important aspects of creating a safe and comfortable sexual environment. Respect means that you understand that everyone has his or her boundaries, desires, and limits when it comes to sex. It also means avoiding any behavior that may make your partner uncomfortable or feel disrespected. Prioritizing respect will help ensure that both partners can fully enjoy themselves during sex without worrying about being violated by their partner's actions or words.

Empathy
Empathy is an important part of creating a safe and comfortable sexual environment. You must try to understand your partner's feelings, desires, and needs. Be attentive to their body language and verbal cues to ensure that they are enjoying themselves and feel comfortable.
Prioritize empathy by asking questions like: "How do you feel about this?" or "Can I do anything differently?"

Education
Before you engage in any sexual activity, it is important to learn about the risks and benefits of that activity. This includes learning about your own body and how it works, as well as what makes other people feel good. For example:
You may want to find out if any health conditions could be exacerbated by certain activities or positions (e.g., arthritis). You could also ask your partner(s) if they have any questions about their bodies or yours--what feels good for them. Where do they like being touched? How much pressure should be applied? This can help ensure that everyone involved is comfortable with what is happening during sex. In addition to learning about each other's bodies and preferences, it's important for both partners not only to know their limits but also respect those limits when making decisions together regarding sexual activities."

Self-Care
Look after your physical and mental health by having enough sleep, eating healthy, and controlling stress. Prioritize your self-care needs so that you can fully enjoy your sexual experiences partner.
Self-care is important for everyone, but especially for people with disabilities who may be more vulnerable to the effects of stress and trauma than others may. Self-care practices such as exercise or meditation can help reduce feelings of isolation and depression, improve sleep quality, and increase energy levels which will improve overall well-being.*

Remember that creating a safe and comfortable sexual environment is a collaborative effort between you and your partner. By prioritizing communication, consent, privacy, protection, comfort, and trust, you can create a space where you can explore your sexuality in a safe and fulfilling way.

CHAPTER SEVEN

Cultivating a Positive Sexual Self-Image

Cultivating a positive sexual self-image can be a difficult, but rewarding journey. It is important to recognize that self-image is often shaped by external influences, like media messages and our personal experiences. It is important to be mindful of the impact these external influences have on our self-image.

As we become more aware of our self-image, we can begin to challenge it. This process involves recognizing our positive and negative internalized beliefs and challenging them. For example, instead of simply believing that "I am not sexually attractive," take the time to explore why this might be so. Is it something that is based on fact, or is it a belief that has been internalized over the years? If it is the latter, can you find ways to challenge and change it?

Part of cultivating a positive sexual self-image is also about exploring our own sexual identities. Who do we find attractive? What kinds of sexual experiences do we want to explore? Taking the time to explore and discover our desires can be a powerful way to help us gain a better understanding and appreciation of our sexuality.

It is important to foster positive relationships with our sexual partners. Open communication and mutual respect are key to creating a healthy and supportive sexual environment. It is also important to recognize that each partner may have different expectations and needs and that it is important to respect these differences.

Cultivating a positive sexual self-image can be difficult, but ultimately rewarding. It involves challenging our own internalized beliefs, exploring our own sexual identity, and fostering positive relationships with our sexual partners. With time, patience, and understanding, we can gain a greater appreciation of our sexuality.

Additionally, there are a few things we can do daily to help cultivate a positive sexual self-image. For starters, taking time to practice self-care is important. This may involve engaging in activities that make us feel good, like going for a walk, reading a book, or taking a hot bath. Additionally, it is also important to recognize body positivity and to take time to practice self-acceptance. This may involve avoiding negative self-talk and instead focusing on the positive aspects of our bodies and sexuality.

It is important to create an environment where we can talk about sex openly and without judgment. Whether it is with friends, family, or a therapist, it is important to have someone to talk to about our own sexual identity and experiences. Doing so can help us feel more empowered and more connected to our sexuality.

Overall, cultivating a positive sexual self-image is an important process that can take time and effort. However, with dedication, understanding, and self-compassion, it is possible to gain a greater appreciation and understanding of our sexuality.

CHAPTER EIGHT

Celebrating Your True Sexuality

Celebrating your true sexuality is all about embracing who you are and what you desire without shame or fear of judgment. It is about owning your sexual identity and finding joy and fulfillment in your sexual experiences.

To celebrate your true sexuality, start by exploring your desires and fantasies in a safe and consensual way. This can include trying new sexual experiences, experimenting with different types of partners, or exploring different types of sexual preferences.

Another way to start celebrating your true sexuality is to create a safe and comfortable environment for yourself. This could involve creating a physical space that is free of judgment or finding activities that make you feel good. Taking time to explore and experiment in ways that feel comfortable and safe is key to celebrating your true sexuality. Additionally, it is also important to create a supportive network of people who can provide a safe space to talk about your sexuality and sexual experiences.

It is also important to communicate your needs and boundaries with your partner(s) and to prioritize your pleasure and satisfaction. This can involve learning to say no when you are not comfortable with something, setting boundaries around what you are willing to do or not do, and advocating for your sexual desires.

To celebrate your true sexuality is to embrace your body and all of its unique features. This can involve practicing self-love and self-care, wearing clothing that makes you feel confident, sexy, and using positive affirmations to boost your self-esteem.

Celebrating your true sexuality can involve being open to trying new things, experimenting, learning from mistakes, and growing from the experience. It is important to remember that sexuality is not a one-size-fits-all experience and that it is okay to explore and learn about what feels most comfortable for you.

Finally, it is important to surround yourself with positive and supportive people who respect and celebrate your sexuality. This can include friends, family, or members of the LGBTQ+ community who share your experiences and can offer support, advice, and encouragement.

Remember, celebrating your true sexuality is a journey, and it is important to be patient, kind, and compassionate with yourself along the way. By embracing whom you are and what you desire, you can live a life filled with joy, pleasure, and fulfillment.

CHAPTER NINE

Overcoming Obstacles

The journey towards self-acceptance can be challenging and often involves overcoming common obstacles that many individuals face. Here are some of the most common obstacles and ways to address them:

Internalized Shame and Guilt:

Many individuals struggle with internalized shame and guilt surrounding their sexuality or other aspects of their identity. To address this, it is important to challenge negative beliefs and replace them with positive affirmations. This may involve working with a therapist or engaging in self-reflection and self-compassion exercises.

Fear of Rejection:

The fear of rejection from family, friends, or society can prevent individuals from fully embracing their true selves. It is important to remember that acceptance from others is not necessary for self-acceptance. Building a support system of individuals who accept and celebrate your true self can also help combat the fear of rejection.

Lack of Role Models:

Many individuals may struggle with self-acceptance due to a lack of representation and role models in media or their personal lives. Seeking out diverse representation and connecting with communities that celebrate and embrace different identities can help combat this obstacle.

Internalized Heteronormativity:

Heteronormative beliefs and expectations can be deeply ingrained in society and individuals, leading to internalized beliefs that conflict with one's true self. To address this, it is important to challenge and question these beliefs and seek out diverse perspectives and resources.

Trauma or Experiences:

Experiences or trauma can affect an individual's journey toward self-acceptance. Seeking out therapy or support groups can help individuals process and heal from these experiences, allowing them to move toward self-acceptance.

It is important to remember that the journey toward self-acceptance is unique for each individual and may involve different obstacles and challenges. However, with patience, self-compassion, and support, individuals can overcome these obstacles and fully embrace their true selves.

Strategies for overcoming these obstacles and finding support

Here are some strategies for overcoming obstacles in the journey toward self-acceptance and finding support:

Seek Professional Help:

Working with a therapist or counselor can provide individuals with tools and strategies to overcome obstacles and work towards self-acceptance.

Connect with Supportive Communities:

Connecting with communities that celebrate and embrace different identities can provide individuals with a sense of belonging and support. This may involve joining online communities, attending support groups, or seeking out local organizations that celebrate diversity.

Practice Self-Care:

Engaging in self-care activities such as meditation, exercise, or creative hobbies can help individuals build resilience and cope with obstacles on the journey toward self-acceptance.

Challenge Negative Beliefs:

Identifying and challenging negative beliefs and replacing them with positive affirmations can help individuals build self-acceptance and self-confidence.

Build a Support System:

Building a support system of friends, family, or allies who accept and celebrate an individual's true self can provide much-needed support and validation.

Educate Yourself:

Seeking out diverse perspectives and resources can help individuals challenge and question internalized beliefs and expand their understanding of different identities and experiences.

Remember that overcoming obstacles on the journey toward self-acceptance takes time, patience, and perseverance. However, with the right tools, strategies, and support, individuals can overcome these obstacles and embrace their true selves.

CHAPTER TEN

Embracing Your True Self

Embracing your true self is a journey that requires self-awareness, self-acceptance, and self-love. It involves recognizing and honoring your unique qualities, strengths, and weaknesses, as well as embracing your sexuality, gender identity, and other aspects of your identity that make you who you are.

Many individuals struggle with self-acceptance due to societal expectations, family beliefs, or personal insecurities. However, embracing your true self is crucial for your mental health, happiness, and overall well-being.

To start embracing your true self, it is important to engage in self-reflection and identify the negative beliefs or thoughts that are holding you back. This may involve challenging societal norms or beliefs that conflict with your identity or values.

Once you have identified these obstacles, it is important to practice self-compassion and kindness towards yourself. This means acknowledging your imperfections and accepting them as a part of who you are.

In addition to self-acceptance, self-care, and self-love are also essential components of embracing your true self. This may involve engaging in activities that bring you joy and fulfillment, surrounding yourself with supportive individuals, and prioritizing your mental and physical health.

Finally, it is important to remember that embracing your true self is an ongoing journey that requires patience and perseverance. It may involve setbacks and challenges, but with self-acceptance, self-love, and support, you can continue to grow and thrive as your authentic self.

www.ingramcontent.com/pod-product-compliance
Lightning Source LLC
Chambersburg PA
CBHW061559250726
48657CB00021B/2404